BALANCED
FAMILY HEALTH
IN AN
UNBALANCED
WORLD

RICHARD L. COMITZ

outskirtspress
DENVER, COLORADO

Outskirts Press, Inc.
http://www.outskirtspress.com

ISBN: 978-1-4787-3779-7

Outskirts Press and the "OP" logo are trademarks belonging to Outskirts Press, Inc.

PRINTED IN THE UNITED STATES OF AMERICA

This book is dedicated to the memory of my father, and to my family. I am blessed to have a supportive family and two awesome children, Hannah, and Louis.

TABLE OF CONTENTS

ACKNOWLEDGMENTS

I would like to thank everyone who has ever touched my life—especially my mother, for being a strong role model. This book would not be possible were it not for my two loving children, Hannah and Louis. Everything I do is with their future in mind.

I would also like to thank the **Institute for Integrative Nutrition™** for flaming the spark that started my passion for a healthier lifestyle.

1
FOREWORD

I first want to provide you with a disclaimer: this book has not been evaluated by the Food and Drug Administration. The information provided here is not intended to diagnose, cure, or prevent any disease, and the recommendations provided herein represent my own personal opinions, based upon my research. Always consult a health care professional with regard to specific questions.

I'd also like to give you a bit of background about where I come from.

I have fond memories of my childhood. I felt that I was in a loving family, and my parents always wanted what was best for us. My mother was a great home-maker who would later work in the food industry. My memories of my father are pleasant, but the picture that sticks in my head is my dad with a large stomach, holding a cigarette. The most impressionable moment of my life was my father's death. He died of cancer when I was just eleven years old. I had to deal with a very tough question: *why our family?*

It seemed that I had to grow up overnight. I was the middle child and the oldest male, so I felt I had to be the man of the house. During the years after my father died, my mother did all she could to provide for us. She quickly progressed from a waitressing job to a managerial position, because she needed the insurance for us along with a better income. My mother did a tremendous job of providing us with a normal upbringing. She was also very successful at her job, rising to the top 15 in her company. With every decision I made, I felt the pressure of doing my best to avoid adding pressure or stress to my mother's already-hectic life. I also felt that my father was always looking down on me, so I wanted to make him proud.

I had a typical high school experience: playing football, running track, and doing my best at my studies. I had thought that I wanted to become a doctor, but I knew medical school was very expensive. I heard of a student who had graduated a few years earlier and entered the United States Military Academy at West

Point. Upon further investigation, I found out that this excellent school actually pays you to attend college in exchange for military service. I figured I would take advantage of this, so I could get my college education paid for. I then had to figure out how to gain admittance to West Point. It turned out to be a difficult process. Faculty members at my high school strongly suggested that I formulate a good Plan B, because most people do not get accepted. This made me work even harder.

I *did* get accepted, and graduated as a member of the class of 1996. Those were some difficult years, but the lessons I learned were invaluable. My thoughts of medical school faded as I struggled just to keep up.

During my time at West Point, I was introduced to my future wife. I still remember coming back to West Point after a weekend home in Pennsylvania, where I had gone on a date with Jadelle. I told my roommate that she was the type of girl I would like to marry. Luckily for me, her feelings were similar. Upon graduation, I was commissioned as a second lieutenant in the Army, and figured I would get out after my five-year commitment. Jadelle and I were married shortly after graduation, and we started our military career together after she graduated from nursing school.

Though there were some difficult times, we found we

really loved the military, especially the people we were blessed to meet. The plan to get out after five years kind of faded away, and as I write this, I am in my 18th year of active-duty service. We have been blessed with two children, Hannah and Louis. They are in my mind with every decision I make, and they are the reason I get up every morning. With all of our moving around, my children have been able to have many experiences most kids don't have access to. I cannot express in words what a positive influence Jadelle has been on their upbringing. Though they are still in middle school and grade school, we can tell that they are destined for greatness in whatever they do.

The choices I have made in my military career have always been carried out with Jadelle's input, and with my family as my first consideration. I have served in many different types of units and at various levels, always enjoying my interactions with people and the challenges facing me. I have been intrigued by the complexity of the world, and with my ability to influence young soldiers and people from other countries. For me, the importance of education and lifelong learning was realized when the Army offered me the chance to get my master's degree and teach at West Pont. Advanced civil schooling gave me the opportunity to stay close to my family and to earn my master's degree, in return for teaching for three years at West Point. Jadelle and I decided to move to sunny Florida, where I attended the Florida Institute of Technology, studying for a Master of Science in Chemistry.

From that point on, I felt I could never read enough or learn enough. I took my job as a teacher and example very seriously. It was important to me to show the cadets what an ideal officer should look like. At West Point, I enjoyed teaching more than I ever could imagine. Later in my career, when the Army offered me the opportunity to get a PhD and teach at West Point again, it was a no-brainer.

Throughout my military career, I have made it a point to stay physically fit and technically and tactically proficient. I figured out what worked for me and my body, and have been able to stay in good physical condition. During my doctoral studies, I realized how important health and nutrition really are. During this time, I celebrated my 36th birthday: the age my father was when he died. I made a commitment to myself not only to be around for my children's lives, but also for their children's children.

At the same time, I chose an original proposal topic and decided to research artificial sweeteners. I learned so much about nutrition and food that my interest continued after the original proposal was finished. I found myself reading about nutrition in all of my free time. I told everyone what I was learning, and made changes in my life that turned out to be very beneficial. I was feeling awesome, and my family was influenced positively, as well. While researching one day, I stumbled upon the Institute of Integrative Nutrition™ and knew that I had to go through the program to become a health coach. Although my military duties represent my primary job, my hobby and passion is to share with as many people as possible what I have learned about leading a balanced, healthy lifestyle.

These days, our world is very unbalanced. The information that we get through the media and commercials is usually funded by big corporations. Even though the science of health has been getting better and better every year, the public has not been given the whole story about nutrition. We have grown into a very unhealthy society, and we have continued to export our unhealthy lifestyle to other countries throughout the world. I felt that writing a book about the entire circle of life would be the best way to communicate what I have learned about nutrition to the largest possible audience. I hope to create a ripple effect, and slowly start changing our unhealthy lifestyle so a greater number of people can live longer, happier lives.

2
INTRODUCTION

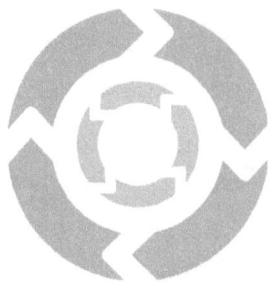

Two major categories can impact your health. I like to use the above graphic to illustrate what I call the inner circle and the outer circle.

The outer circle represents everything you do with your body, and the environment outside of your physical self. We will go into this in great detail in the next chapter, but for now, the outer circle will encompass relationships, physical environment, career, physical fitness, stress, friends, etc.

The inner circle represents everything you put into your body. This primarily includes food, but also skin care products and other such things. The two circles are linked by knowledge, motivation, and awareness.

Balancing the two circles is probably the most challenging part of life. It should be obvious that both areas feed your total health, and cannot be mutually exclusive. Even if you are doing everything in a balanced way with regard to the outer circle, if you are not feeding your inner circle correctly, you can still be unhealthy. Likewise, if you are feeding your body the most nutritious foods, but are in a hostile relationship, you will not be healthy, either. It takes knowledge and awareness to make adjustments to either or both of these circles. That's where this book comes in. I will give you the knowledge, but it is up to you to be aware of what affects your health the most. You must then have the courage to make positive changes on your own.

Looking at the image a little more closely, you can see that the first figure represents an individual. It is shown by itself in order to illustrate the points simply, but in fact, a person can never exist as a single circle. Your outer circle is irrevocably linked to other people in your life. When you are growing up, it contains family members, friends, teachers, etc.; but when you start a relationship, you link your outer circle with that of your significant other. For simplicity's sake, it would look like the figure at the left, below.

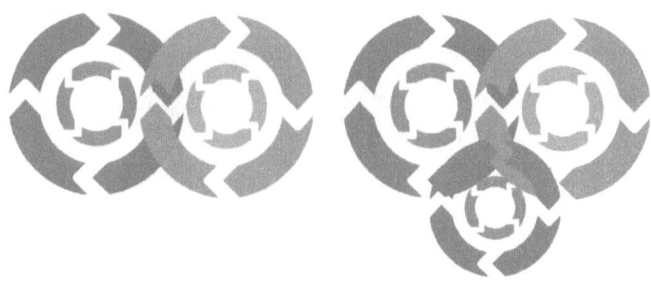

One can imagine that if two people have a child (whether through natural childbirth or adoption), the result would look like the figure at right, above. I think you can understand the idea that your outer circle is linked to many others. This is how one person can affect another. If you think about it, this is a very powerful concept. If you can figure out which outer-circle links are negatively contributing to your health, you can change them through awareness, taking steps to gain the knowledge and make a positive change.

This book focuses upon family health. Because we have to start somewhere, we will start from the time a young adult meets the person they want to spend the rest of their life with. I recognize, as you should, that through self-awareness, you may find that you cannot be healthy until you take care of the part of your outer circle that originated in your early years. When starting a new relationship, however, you are consciously connecting your outer circle to someone else's. Additionally, when you make positive linkages with others, you will crowd out any negative linkages.

From the time you meet your soul mate, you should both consider your long-term health and wellness together. Your happiness will become contagious, and your healthy lifestyle will influence others to improve their own. All of your decisions, from this point forward, should be a collaborative effort. Remember to continually appreciate and support each other. Throughout your life together, many life changes will occur that you will have to take on. It is much easier to face challenges when you are both optimally healthy. When the time is right to welcome children into your life, you will then have to consider their future health, as well.

The most important thing you can do, next to taking care of yourself, is to take care of your children. We will spend several chapters discussing key periods in their development and how you can contribute to their health. They will be watching your example from the first time they set eyes upon you. Though loving your child is essential, love does not mean you can let them do or have whatever they want. Teaching them good habits early on will pay off for the rest of their lives. Teaching them that hard work, discipline, dedication, and compassion are woven into their fabric will influence their appropriate actions at all times; and when they slip up, you will be there to love them and set them back on course. At some point, they will grow old enough to no longer need as much guidance. This is when you can step back—but always be there when they need someone to talk to.

There will come a point when your children will leave your home, and go out on their own. You should feel confident that they are prepared to take on life as adults. You have been preparing them for this all of their lives. You and your spouse will be left alone. Although it is difficult to stay completely connected to your spouse during the early childhood years—because you are taking kids to soccer practice and everything else in their busy lives—it is always important to appreciate your spouse and maintain your health. Now, when the kids are out on their own, you should make it a point to really improve and nurture your relationship with your spouse. This will help you continue to be a positive influence upon those around you, and keep you in strong form for your adult children.

Soon, grandchildren will come along. These times can be both joyous and challenging to your health. If you have prepared by keeping yourself healthy, you will be able to keep up with your grandchildren, both physically and mentally. The challenging part will be recognizing that your children have to make their own decisions about how to raise their children. It will have been many years since you have raised a small child, and things will have changed.

Consider my example: when I was a child, computers took up a whole room, and phones were mounted on the wall. Now, you can carry your computer around and call from a cell phone anywhere, anytime. Even with technology and everything that comes with it, you still have to be there for your children. They will need someone to talk to about raising children, and this is the time when listening will be more important that offering advice.

During your final days, the most important life events to look back upon will be your relationships. You will be able to live your last few days in peace, knowing that you were loved and that people knew you loved them in return. You will know that you did all you could, and will have no regrets.

The next three chapters are probably the most important in the book. They will give you a baseline of knowledge for making decisions that will keep your outer and inner circles equally healthy. They will also provide tips for keeping both of these areas balanced in our unbalanced world. With this information, you will have the tools to lead a healthy life. You will then be ready to join your outer circle with your significant other, and start a whole new chapter in your balanced existence.

3
OUTER CIRCLE

This is the first of the two key areas that contribute greatly to your overall health. The outer circle is not typically considered when we refer to health, but in many cases, it turns out to be just as important as the foods you eat. The outer circle involves many aspects of your life, which will be covered in this chapter along with tips and tools for improving these areas.

Your personal outlook functions as the lens through which you view everything in your life. You can choose to be a glass-half-full or a glass-half-empty type of person. It really *is* that simple: YOU can choose. I am sure that if I asked you which type of person is healthier, you would respond with glass-half-full: so why not start trying to be more positive in your view of life right now?

More and more people tend to worry about what others are doing, or what other people have, and become jealous. Jealousy, selfishness, pride, and greed reside at the center of most disputes. If people could just focus upon their own lives and always find something to be thankful for, we would have less conflict. If you maintain a positive outlook, and feel happy for others when they are fortunate, you tend to face your own adversity better. Instead of looking for someone else to blame, just take personal responsibility. With a positive attitude, you are freed to make a whole range of changes to better yourself.

I am the type of person who believes that everything happens for a reason. If this is true, then it is not worth getting upset when things don't go your way. You will still have to deal with whatever the situation is, so why not do it in a positive manner? This will influence the attitudes of people around you, as well. Think of someone who is a glass-half-empty type of person. How does it feel to be around that person? Are other people around them happy?

Being negative, mad, or upset all the time has an effect on your physical health, as well. Your heart rate and blood pressure become elevated when you are angry. Over time, these continual physical stressors can lead to a heart attack or stroke. Learning to deal with adversity with a level head and positive attitude will always result in a healthier life.

Confidence is the character trait that will most help you to succeed. It is imperative that you remain confident that you can accomplish whatever task you set out to do. This will also enhance your personal outlook. Doubt in yourself leaves room for failure. Fear of failure is the reason why many people do not attempt something important to them, or quit before completing the task. A lack of confidence in yourself will be very apparent to others. In the long term, it can affect not only your physical health, but the health of those around you, as well.

One of the biggest stressors on self-confidence is other people. Whether it is someone saying you cannot succeed, or ridiculing you for a minor setback, it can result in you shutting down or not trying. It becomes crucial that you evaluate your outer circle, and surround yourself with people who truly believe in you. It may also be helpful to remember that many people have failed, but have gone on to become very successful, because they were confident that they could do it.

President Abraham Lincoln stands as a perfect example. He failed in business, and was defeated in elections for state legislature, Senate, Congress, and Vice President. He also lost his sweetheart, and experienced a nervous breakdown. Eventually, though, he became one of our best presidents. In today's world, inspirational people such as wounded veterans have bounced back from the adversity of losing a limb with absolute confidence that they would walk again. Whenever you are doubting yourself, realize that someone worse off has been able to overcome adversity—and so can you.

Stress comes as the result of allowing your outer circle to inflict undue pressure upon you. It usually results from imbalance in some part of your life. This is a good time to discuss balance in a little more depth. Balance stems from the ability to allot an appropriate amount of time and effort to the many activities and people most important to you on a daily basis. A simple example could be illustrated in a person who has work, a spouse, a child, and church group to attend to. All of these elements are important, but it's easy to see what would happen to their health if an imbalance were to arise between, say, work and their child. If someone spent so much time at work that they never saw their child, this could greatly impact their health due to the stress of not being there when their child needed them.

Conversely, if they took too much time off from work in order to spend more with their child, their productivity could suffer, and stress could arise from a boss or manager. The ability to balance all of the people and activities in your life is very challenging, but probably represents the single most important area for limiting the effects of stress on your health.

Since stress is one of the major outer-circle contributors to poor health, it becomes very important to have effective means at your disposal for releasing tension and coping with stress so that it does not end up adversely affecting your life. First, evaluate your goals and priorities to ensure you are focusing your effort in the right areas. Even the most balanced people experience stress, so it is important to have ready outlets to relieving it. Talking with others, exercise, and hobbies are just a few ways to deal with and release stress.

The ways we entertain ourselves can also play an important role in our overall health. One could think of many activities that contribute to a poor sense of well-being. If you are staying up late at night to watch TV or surf the Internet at the cost of precious sleep, you could be hurting your health more than you know. Sleep is crucial to good health, and serves as a time when your body can recharge. If you are continually deprived of adequate sleep, it could affect your long-term health and longevity.

In the same vein, if you are going out several nights a week, you may not be getting adequate sleep—not to mention that the bar or nightclub environment usually brings out pressure to smoke and/or drink excessive alcohol. You may also be subjected to secondhand smoke. As we will discover in the inner-circle portion of the book, alcohol really has no nutritional value, so if you do decide to drink, you should do so in moderation.

My recommendation for entertainment would be to choose activities that allow you to interact with the people you care about. Whether it's a movie or dinner, you benefit from positive social interactions. You can also try activities that are physically and/or mentally stimulating. Anytime you exercise your brain and/or body, you are contributing to your good health. You can also turn to a hobby: projects or activities that give you something to work at or look forward to completing.

Relationships represent a crucial part of your outer circle. Positive relationships with people contribute greatly to your good health, along with friends who support you and can be honest with you. In many cases, people carry negative influences in their outer circle. An abusive or unsupportive person can really drive you to poor health.

Family relationships are a double-edged sword. Family members can act as the most supportive presences in our lives, or represent the reason for deep emotional problems. It is very hard to deal with family members who are negatively impacting your health. You must find you own personal way to deal with these people. Because they are family, it is often best just to be cordial, and avoid sharing large amounts of information.

Another relationship that is often overlooked is the one you have with your pet. If you care for an animal, you can usually see their unconditional love for you. You, in turn, feel obligated to feed them, exercise them, and love them back. This is a positive environment, and usually contributes positively to your health, as well.

Your career represents the context in which you spend a large part of your life, so if you are unhappy in your job, it can have a drastic effect on your health. From the time you start thinking about a career, consider the options you like and that would provide you with the lifestyle you desire. In some cases, things happen that stop our initial dreams from coming to fruition. At this point, people will usually take a job that pays the bills, but does not provide much in the way of personal satisfaction. It is important to find strategies to get through this time in your life; persist in your search for a job that is satisfying to you.

The environment at your job site can also exert a huge impact on your health. If you are working in your chosen profession and have a terrible boss or coworkers, your health could still suffer. It is imperative not to settle for anything less than a satisfying job and positive work environment. If you are not able to get there immediately, take steps to get there. Being productive and doing something you love will greatly contribute to positive health and well-being.

Financial concerns are usually tied to your job, as well. We often find ourselves looking at what other people have, and think we deserve the same. Living within our means is something that doesn't always seem normal anymore. Many people turn to credit to get what they want rather than what they actually need for survival. We have to get past the idea that material items make us happy. I suggest writing down a budget and sticking to it. In your budget, include daily expenditures, entertainment, long-term savings, and short-term savings.

Learning to stick to a budget will alleviate quite a bit of stress later on.

Whether you are religious or not, your life should contain some sense of spirituality. When considering this area of your life, some of the more well-known religions commonly come to mind. Each tradition includes a sense of belonging and the means to ask for forgiveness, both of which are very important when trying to improve your health. Religion usually provides a way of showing acceptance, and recognizes that we are all human and make mistakes. The "rules" represent boundaries and objectives to try to live up to.

If you do not identify with any one religion, it is still important to cultivate a sense of spirituality. Spirituality can be defined as a sense of a deeper meaning or value. If your worldview does not include religion, you should still provide yourself with a way to feel and comprehend the essence of life. Spirituality can be accessed through meditation, prayer, or contemplation; but whichever route you decide to take, you must have access to relaxation and reflection.

Some of the most innocent and fulfilling times in my life happened simply when I was outside. Take time to appreciate how much better you feel when you can breathe fresh air and feel the rays of the sun. The sight of the different colors and shapes of nature have the power to bring a smile to our faces, or bring back a good memory. Savor these moments, and you will feel better instantly.

Unfortunately, numerous toxins and pollutants are present in our environment. Humans spray pesticides and insecticides. We also clean and coat the surfaces that we touch daily with potentially toxic substances. This is not mentioned to make you paranoid—just aware. If you develop or already have a chronic issue that cannot be explained by anything else, you may want to look at your environment. You can make subtle changes, and see how your issue improves or gets worse, accordingly.

Along with the products we use to clean our clothes and homes, we must also consider what we clean our bodies with. Many of the chemicals in our personal skin care products can contribute to long-term, detrimental health effects. Let's examine a few key chemicals you should try to reduce in your life, along with their potential side effects. They are listed on the environmental working group website (EWG.org). I encourage you to do your own research in this area.

Parabens are usually present in soaps, creams, and make-up. They have similar structures, and act as hormone disruptors. They have also been found in breast cancer cells.

Methylchloroisothiazlinone is an allergen and harmful to the nervous system.

PEG (polyethylene glycol), dioxane, and *TEA (triethanolamine)* are chemicals in shampoo, hairspray, and skin creams. They are allergens, and have been linked to cancer.

Sodium lauryl or *laureth sulfate* is found in shampoo and detergents. This additive can cause damage to skin and adverse reactions.

Triclosan is in antibacterial soap and hand sanitizer. Besides damaging the environment, it is a thyroid disruptor, dries the skin, and has been linked to muscle weakness.

Oxybenzone and *cinnamates* may damage cell protein and DNA. They have also been found to disrupt hormones.

Glycolic, AHA and *BHA* acids are contained in many anti-aging products. They cause increased photosensitivity, irritation, and possible permanent skin damage.

The research available improves every day, and you should always continue to check your products. I am not saying that you should throw everything out; but I am suggesting you use the products with the fewest possible side effects. The fact is, we are just now finding out about the long-term effects of ingredients we put in products 20 years ago. Lastly, remember that manufacturers are usually in the business of making money, and often do not look out for our best interest. We are the only ones who can do that.

Exercise may represent the most important portion of your outer circle. I like to think of exercise as a way to ensure that I am able to keep up with my children and their children. The better shape you keep yourself in now, the more agile you will be as you grow older. You will be less of a burden on others as you get older, and more importantly, you will be able to continue to enjoy your life longer.

Exercise helps control weight, but please don't believe that just because you exercise, you can eat whatever you want. To put this into perspective, if you want to exercise off one pound, you have to burn 3500 calories;

and by the way, running for 30 minutes burns about 350 calories. Not too many people have the time to do that much exercise. Exercise represents a part of maintaining and/or losing weight, but only one component. Here are some benefits of exercise, as referenced from the Mayo Clinic.

Exercise gets your blood pumping and stresses your body's systems in a good way. No matter what your current weight, being active boosts high-density lipoprotein (HDL) or "good" cholesterol, and decreases unhealthy triglycerides. This combination keeps your blood flowing smoothly, which decreases your risk of cardiovascular disease. In fact, regular physical activity can help you prevent or manage a wide range of health problems and concerns, including stroke, metabolic syndrome, type 2 diabetes, depression, certain types of cancer, arthritis, and falls.

Your mood and energy levels can be improved by exercise, as well. Physical activity stimulates various brain chemicals that can leave you feeling happier and more relaxed. You may also feel better about your appearance when you exercise regularly; it can boost your confidence and improve your self-esteem.

Exercise improves your muscle strength and boosts your endurance. Exercise and physical activity deliver oxygen and nutrients to your tissues and help your cardiovascular system work more efficiently. When your heart and lungs work more easily, you have more energy to go about your daily chores. As a bonus, you usually sleep better, too!

Finally, exercise is a great way to clear your mind and reduce stress. No matter how busy your life is, you should try to incorporate about 30 minutes of exercise into your day, at least five times per week. You should intentionally put exercise into your schedule, and dedicate yourself to getting it done. You can be creative about how you fit it exercise in. Whether you choose to take a class, walk, run, bike, weight train, or play sports…just get out there!

4
INNER CIRCLE

It is estimated that ninety percent of all diseases, disorders, and aliments can be prevented, managed, or cured by what we eat. Your nutrition represents the most important way to improve your day-to-day performance and attitude. There is no one-size-fits-all prescription for nutrition. It is different for everyone, but there are definitely some common guidelines that will help everyone stay healthy.

If you feel like you have a long way to go in this category, just take it slowly. The best way to make healthy changes is to crowd out unhealthy foods with healthy foods. I promise you, over time, these healthy choices will stay in your life, and you will not even know why you ate any other way. You may have to unlearn some things that you have come to believe about nutrition that may not necessarily be true. This section will cover the general trends and recommendations about how to crowd out unhealthy choices. It will also give you tips on how to read labels, shop, and prepare foods. Finally, we'll briefly address some dietary changes to help discover if food sensitivities or allergies are causing poor health.

Before we start looking specifically at nutrition, I want to bring some facts to the forefront about what our society has taught us. Without getting too political, just understand that government recommendations are usually made with industries in mind more than your personal health. Do your own research when it comes to government regulations. For example, the United States Department of Agriculture makes recommendations for food intake, but they are also charged with promoting agricultural interests. Also, the Food and Drug Administration will allow chemicals to pass as "generally regarded as safe" if no major, readily apparent negative effects exist. Unfortunately, no matter how well-intentioned they are, they do not have their own independent scientists to verify everything that is introduced to the market. In addition, the FDA does not carry out regular reviews of chemicals that were approved many years ago.

Research and scientific knowledge continue to get better and better every year. We are now finding out that things we have believed to be true for many years may not be exactly correct. One example can be seen in fat content in food. Back in the 1980s, we recognized the increase in heart disease, and were looking for a culprit. Researchers saw a relationship linking fat to heart disease, so we started taking the fat out of all of our foods. The problem was that fat was usually replaced with sugar to ensure that the food still tasted good. We now know that the *type* of fat consumed is more important. There are many benefits to healthy fats, which we will discuss later in this chapter. The low-fat craze did not work, because heart disease is still rising. There is a great deal of research out now pointing to the negative effects of sugar.

The final point I would like to make is about media and advertising. We are continually bombarded with food ads and commercials. Foods are packaged in bright colors, and use specific words to attract certain audiences. For example, children's foods are packaged in primary colors with mascots on the front, and for parents, they are labeled as healthy. Other foods are marketed as healthy via wording on the package, but the ingredients are not that good. Unfortunately, there is little advertising or marketing for genuinely healthy foods. Remember, food makers and distributors are in the business of making a profit, so they will do whatever is necessary to accomplish that. This means it will be important to pay particular attention the section in this chapter about reading labels.

The first aspect of your nutrition you should take a look at is what you are drinking. These days, we have so many choices about what to drink, but the sad reality is that most of the choices are not good ones. My first recommendation is to try to drink a lot more water. Try to replace what you are currently drinking during your day with water. Our bodies are 75% water, so this is what we need to allow for normal body function. Although other beverages are also liquid, they cannot hydrate your body like water can.

I don't want this to be all about what *not* to do, but I do want to tell you why what you drink may not be contributing to a healthy diet. A low-fat milk free of artificial hormones is good for growing. This is why milk is suggested for children. It is also the reason you really do not need it that much when you are an adult. Some people believe that too much milk intake as an adult will just feed bad things in your body, such as tumors.

Juices are one of those things we grew up thinking were very good for us. Juices certainly have their benefits, but should not be your primary drink. It is much better to get your fruit juice along with the fiber in the actual fruit. Fruit juices tend to contain quite a bit of sugar, which will quickly get to your liver and overwhelm the mitochondria's ability to use it efficiently, forcing your body to store some of the calories as fat.

Coffee and tea feature benefits and drawbacks. If you drink them without adding sweeteners, they are a low-calorie drink; but if you get them from popular coffee shops, they are probably not very healthy. I would also rather that you drink coffee or tea because you enjoy them, not because you need them to function in the morning. Caffeine has been shown to have both positive and negative effects on your health. The best choice would be to drink these beverages in moderation.

Sport and energy drinks have become increasingly popular. They are usually filled with extra sugar, artificial sweeteners, and artificial colors. As far as energy drinks go, you should strive to increase your energy through your diet, not through an artificial boost of sugar and caffeine. My recommendation is to phase these out. Sports drinks are meant for athletes. If you are a marathon runner or professional football player, you could drink Gatorade during or immediately after performing, but most of us are not elite athletes. The fact is, the amount of sugar in the drinks outweighs the other benefits. I would phase these out, as well.

Of all available mainstream drinks, soda probably has the biggest negative impact on our society's health. It is filled with processed sugar, artificial sweeteners, and artificial colors. As was discussed with fruit juice, soda dumps a lot of sugar into our systems at one time. Our liver cannot handle this much sugar, so it eventually turns into fat. Sugar and artificial sweeteners do not signal to our brains that we have had enough, so we tend to drink more. You should definitely try to eliminate soda from your diet. I will discuss some of the science about sugar, artificial sweeteners, and artificial color later in this chapter.

Fruits and vegetables are probably the most underrepresented foods in our modern diet, and they are full of valuable minerals, vitamins, and phytochemicals. They also have been linked to the prevention of many diseases and disorders. Whole fruits and vegetables include high levels of fiber, which aids healthy digestion. Folate is crucial to fetal development. Potassium is involved in many cell functions, and helps regulate blood pressure. Vitamin A promotes healthy eyes and skin; thiamin and riboflavin assist in turning food into energy. Vitamin B6 helps in the creation of healthy cells. Vitamin C aids in healing; Vitamin E helps maintain healthy cells. Iron and vitamin K strengthen our blood. Calcium helps build strong bones and assists with cellular signaling. Zinc promotes growth and boosts the immune system. Phytochemicals prevent diseases. The list goes on and on!

Most people probably already know that fruits and vegetables provide incredible benefits; the key is to figure out how to add more of them to your diet. Try new fruits and vegetables at every opportunity! You may have to try something a number of times in order to get a taste for it. Try to prepare vegetables in many different ways in order to find the best options for you. Soups are a great way to get more vegetables. Try to increase the amount of salads you eat, as well. Fruits and vegetables are also great snacks. Shop for what is in season. Seasonal fruits and vegetables are usually cheaper and fresher, so the chance of finding something that tastes good is increased. In summary, if you make any change to your diet, it should be to include more fruits and vegetables.

Protein is a very necessary part of the diet. It is important because it contains the essential building blocks—amino acids—that comprise everything in our bodies, from hair to muscle. About half of the protein goes to making enzymes, which in turn are responsible for catalyzing reactions promoting normal function.

Most of us grew up thinking that you have to eat meat for protein, but this is not entirely true. Many sources of protein exist that do not fall into the category of meat, and still give your body the necessary protein and amino acids to function appropriately. I encourage you to try to vary the sources of your protein.

The major sources of protein will be discussed in this section. Lean beef, such as 97% ground beef, is an excellent source of zinc, iron, and vitamin B12. On the negative side, it has more saturated fat than other protein sources. Buffalo (bison) represents a good beef substitute. It usually costs more, but it is lower in fat and higher in protein. Many healthful diets do not advocate beef. My recommendation is to eat it in moderation, and avoid making it a meal option every night. Eating beef once or twice a week, in my opinion, is not bad.

Poultry includes chicken, turkey, and other birds. White meat is better than dark meat, because dark meat contains more fat. When preparing poultry, be sure to remove the skin. Also, baking is always better than frying.

Pork tenderloin is a very good lean meat, as well. You could probably guess that frying is bad, but covering your meat in too many sauces also detracts from its nutritional benefits. Try to limit your pork to baked tenderloin.

Seafood offers many benefits to your health, above and beyond protein content. Fish is usually higher in the "good" fats—omega-3 fatty acids—which, researchers are finding, are very good for many bodily systems and work to defend against various diseases. Fish also tends to be very lean, so the more fish you can eat, the better off you'll be.

Dairy will be discussed in a section of its own, and represents an excellent source of protein, calcium, and vitamin D in your diet.

Eggs can be selected as one of the cheapest forms of protein. A few years ago, there was a bit of a stir about the cholesterol in egg yolks, but this is really not an issue for most people. Egg whites contain much of the available protein, but the yolks unlock vitamin D and other essential nutrients.

One-half cup of beans contains as much protein as an ounce of steak, without the saturated fats—making beans an excellent protein source to add to your diet. They act as very versatile side dishes, and can even be served as main dishes. Beans are also loaded with fiber, which is helpful in digestion and maintaining normal function.

As far as benefits go, nuts are on the same level as beans, and they are great for snacks on the go. Many people are allergic to certain types of nuts, so if you notice any kind of change after eating nuts, you should see a doctor.

Soy has been linked to heart health. It has also been shown to reduce cholesterol. This is a very versatile source of protein, and many vegetarians use it as a major part of their diet. Tofu is produced from soy, and can be used in an infinite number of dishes, from entrees to desserts. When shopping for soy, be sure to buy organic; soy is one of the main genetically modified crops in this country.

Don't forget that many vegetables also contain protein: peas, spinach, and broccoli, to name just a few. If you are trying to subtly change your diet, don't worry that just because you are not eating meat at every meal, you are not getting enough protein. Simply choose your vegetables wisely.

Many other sources of protein exist that I have not yet mentioned here. Certain grains contain significant amounts of protein, along with many foods from the Asian diet that have now become more mainstream and readily available in the U.S. Do your own research; don't be afraid of trying new things. The most important key, which I will continue to emphasize, is variety in your protein sources. Eat what makes you feel healthy. The ideal protein source—the one that makes you feel best—is different for everyone, and you will actually feel better than usual when you eat protein that is right for you.

Starch represents a category you may need to relearn. In the last 20 or so years, we have associated starch with carbohydrates, and we were told that carbohydrates make you gain weight. This is not exactly true. As with the other categories, it is your *selection* of starches that dictates whether your body uses it for good or bad. One quick example that works to dispel the myth that carbohydrates cause weight gain can be observed in the Japanese diet, which consists of whole grain rice, vegetables, and fish. No obesity problems arise when following a Japanese diet.

It is important to select healthy starches. What you want to look for is whole grains. Any other grains are automatically stripped of their nutrients. You will sometimes see "enriched flour" in an ingredients list, which simply means that the grain has been stripped of its nutrition, with some of the nutrients put back in after that process. It is essential that you read labels carefully and eat whole grains, including brown rice, whole wheat bread, and many others. Look at the label, and make sure you notice two or more grams of fiber. This will tell you that you are getting good grains. Some people will argue that grains are not important, and others that will argue that they are. Listen to your body. Some people really feel they need grains, and others do not.

This is a good time to bring up gluten, a protein found in wheat and related grains. Some people are severely allergic to gluten. This is called Celiac disease. People who have Celiac disease experience adverse reactions to gluten, which can run the gamut of symptoms in terms of severity. In addition, an increasing amount of research points to gluten sensitivity. These people may not experience severe effects like someone with Celiac disease. Many people do not even know that they have a gluten sensitivity, which can manifest itself differently in each person. If you have a chronic, unexplainable health issue like headaches, bloating, an irritated digestive system, or diarrhea, a gluten-free diet may help you. There is also research linking gluten to Attention Deficit Disorder. If something is not going right with your body, try looking at your diet.

Dairy includes such things as milk, yogurt, and cheese. The benefits of low-fat dairy include high levels of protein, calcium, magnesium, folate, B1, B2, B6, B12, and vitamins A, D, and E. It is very good for growth, so children should eat dairy if they are not allergic to it. An increasing number of people say that dairy is not necessary for an adult diet. Simply listen to your body. I would recommend that as you get older and stop growing, you should try to slow down your dairy intake.

Dairy represents another commonly allergenic food, often causing reactions in people with lactose intolerance. Lactose intolerance can result in gas, belly pain, or bloating. It comes as the result of the small intestine failing to produce sufficient *lactase*, which breaks down the sugar *lactose*. Lactose intolerance can manifest itself later in life, or after a digestive problem, so be aware that it is not necessarily something you are born with. Consider removing dairy from your diet if you feel adverse effects after consuming it.

Fat has gotten a bad reputation in the last 20 or so years. When we saw an increase in heart disease in the 1980s, we linked it to fat. Well, that was only partially correct, but it didn't matter: we all grew up thinking if we ate fat, we would gain weight. The key here is the type of fat. The fats to avoid are called *trans fats* (partially hydrogenated oils) and saturated fats. They are usually found in processed foods, are linked to elevated cholesterol levels, and can lead to heart disease and stroke.

More recent research has shown that good, unsaturated fats help fight the very diseases that consuming excess fat was said to cause. Unsaturated fats are divided into *monounsaturated fats* and *polyunsaturated fats*, and both types are thought to impart beneficial effects in terms of healthy cholesterol levels. Monounsaturated fats help lower LDL (bad) cholesterol while also boosting HDL (good) cholesterol. Polyunsaturated fats are also thought to help lower both total and bad cholesterol. Monounsaturated fats tend to be favored over polyunsaturated fats, however, because some research suggests that polyunsaturated fats are less stable, and can reduce levels of good cholesterol as well as bad. Let's not ignore polyunsaturated fats, though. They represent excellent sources of omega-3 fatty acids, which are found mostly in fish, nuts, oils and seeds, but also in dark leafy greens, flaxseed oils, and some vegetable oils. One type of omega-3, *essential fatty acids*, cannot be manufactured independently by our bodies, so consuming these nutrients is the only way to get them. Omega-3 fatty acids are thought to lower blood pressure, combat LDL (bad) cholesterol, fight inflammation, and protect the brain and nervous system.

The last category to consider with regard to overall health impact is sweets. I think everyone knows that they should reduce the amount of sweets they eat. I never say never when it comes to sweets; just be aware that you don't need dessert every meal. It is probably best to make it the high point of your week, and something to look forward to. If you do choose to indulge, do so just a few times a week. Less is better, but never change your diet so much that you are unhappy. By following some of the recommendations in this book, you will probably crave sweets less than you have in the past.

Let's take a closer look at sugar. I will get a little more scientific here, but I think this is necessary for a full understanding of its effects. Sugar, whether in the form of honey, molasses, high-fructose corn syrup, or any other sweet, is really the same at the molecular level. All are mainly sucrose.

Sucrose is a disaccharide that has one glucose molecule connected to one fructose molecule. Once ingested, a disaccharide breaks up into two sugars. Right off the bat, 80% of the glucose gets used by the body, whereas only about 20% of the fructose gets used by the body. The remainder of both go to the liver. The liver processes glucose and fructose differently. Glucose is used as necessary, and less of it tends to be stored as fat. Fructose stresses more of the liver systems, and results in high uric acid levels, more fat deposits, and increased LDL (bad fat). These results exacerbate the symptoms of metabolic syndrome. Fructose does not trigger the release of hormones, such as *insulin* and *leptin*, properly. This results in an absence of feeling full, so you end up eating more than you need to. If you can decrease the amount of added sugar you take in, it will help your overall health tremendously. The problem is that sugar is in everything, so you really have to read the labels.

The next logical question is: what about artificial sweeteners? Well, although the Food and Drug Administration categorizes them as "generally regarded as safe," research shows that they may have serious adverse effects. Artificial sweeteners have been associated with a whole range of severe problems, from headaches to death. Many people do not associate artificial sweeteners with ailments such as headaches or depression, but these additives can cause symptoms without you even knowing it. The problem is that they break down into metabolites, which can disrupt the chemical equilibrium in the body—especially in the area of the brain associated with behavior. Artificial sweeteners are added to many things without your knowledge. You may think you are making good choices, and still find out that your product contains an artificial sweetener that is causing a health problem. Mounting research shows that artificial sweeteners do not do what they are advertised to do, which is to help you lose weight. Listed below are the common artificial sweeteners, along with some of the problems that have been associated with them.

Acesulfame potassium (or K) has mostly been shown to leave the body intact, but anyone who has a sulfa allergy could experience adverse effects. Some people may not realize they have a sulfa allergy, and the resulting symptoms can be confused with other problems.

Aspartame, for me, is the sweetener with the greatest number of problems associated with it. Structurally, it is very similar to *neotame*. They both contain metabolites that can affect the part of the brain related to behavior.

Saccharin has been shown in studies to leave the body mostly intact. There are also studies that show it breaks down into other metabolites. These metabolites can cause adverse effects, such as depression.

Sucralose has been found to damage the good bacteria and microflora in the digestive system. With long-term use, it can lead to an irritated digestive system.

Many other sweeteners are also emerging on the market, such as *stevia*. Manufacturers are always looking for sweeteners that taste good and have no calories. I would imagine that even more will come out after this book is published. Here's the key to remember: if sweeteners are pure and from nature, I would not really argue against them, but once they have been processed, I would avoid them. Industry has a history of taking something good and refining it into something bad. No matter what your sweetener of choice, simply use less of it, and soon you will no longer crave it.

The bottom line is that all sweeteners are artificial to our bodies. We all deal with them differently, but if you can avoid sweeteners, I would suggest it. I feel very strongly about not giving artificial sweeteners to pregnant women or children. I believe that the developing brain could be negatively affected by artificial sweeteners, and that the related metabolites could be associated with conditions on the autism spectrum or with other behavioral disorders. Artificial sweeteners have also been tied to depression, and can significantly alter mood. For me, too much evidence points to the negative effects of artificial sweeteners to take a chance.

The same arguments can be made for artificial colors, which can occur in any color number combination found in an ingredient list, such as red 40. Their metabolites are surprisingly similar to artificial sweetener metabolites, and can impact the part of the brain responsible for behavior. Many groups say that artificial colors are the cause of autism and behavioral disorders, along with depression and mood problems. There are no known positive results of eating red- or blue-colored foods. They are usually dyed to attract children and to make things look better, but they do not affect taste. Many products are now coming out with coloring that is not artificial, such as beet juice. I would suggest trying to select these choices, instead.

Another artificial practice we are learning more about is introduction of genetically modified organisms (GMOs) into our food supply. GMOs could be present in fruits, vegetables, grain, and/or meat. Research has been showing more and more that these types of foods may be the cause of many of the diseases and disorders we suffer from today. You can do more research on this if you like, but I would try to stay away from GMO foods, as well. It is difficult to be sure you are avoiding GMOs because currently there are no requirements to label foods that contain GMOs so do your research. The main crops affected by genetic modification are corn, soy, potatoes, and canola; try to buy organic, instead, and watch out for hidden soy in ingredient lists.

I would like to give you some additional information to help you sort through food labels. Most of the time, a better alternative exists to most of the foods you like. I have five simple tips to use while shopping for foods. They are recommended by Dr. David L. Katz of Yale University, in his *Nutrition Detectives* program.

- Do not be fooled by anything the front of a package says. The bright colors and words are just meant to attract you to the product, regardless of actual content. You should turn to the nutrition portion of the package immediately.

- The first ingredient is always present in highest quantity in the product. If it is sugar, you are probably not doing well in selecting this item.

- Avoid partially hydrogenated oils and high-fructose corn syrup (or any other added sugar, by any alias).

- Avoid foods with long ingredient lists. If you cannot identify most of the ingredients, you probably should not choose this food.

- Find whole grains, and look for at least two grams of fiber.

Other general tips for shopping include buying your food locally, which ensures freshness and limits processing. In addition, shopping the perimeter of the grocery store (the fresh, perishable items) is much better than shopping the interior of the grocery store (the shelves, which contain preserved, processed foods). I would recommend non-GMO, organic fruits and vegetables, because they are free of chemicals such as pesticides and herbicides; but at the very least, make every effort to start eating more fruits and vegetables in general.

As far as food preparation goes, I would suggest trying to eat fruits and vegetables raw whenever possible. Most people know they should skip fried food. Try many different methods of preparing food, and try to enhance flavor with natural spices. Pay attention to portion control, as we usually eat too much, too fast. Have fun, and don't be afraid to experiment!

Finally, carry out your own research about what science says is good for you to eat. Right now, things we have not heard of before are showing promising results for enhanced health. Take a look at chia seeds, quinoa, oats, pumpkin, and kale. Remember, you can't go wrong by increasing your fruit and vegetable consumption.

5
LINKAGES

Knowledge, awareness, and motivation create healthy linkages between your outer circle and inner circle. These are the mechanisms by which you can successfully adjust your lifestyle. So many people who want to make lifestyle changes find themselves able to grasp one or two of the linkages; but it isn't until they comprehend all three that they can make real changes. All are interconnected, and together, they contribute to improving your overall health.

The first and most difficult element, for many people, is awareness. It can be hard for many of us to perform an honest assessment of our general health, and it is even harder to identify the habits, activities, or routines that are actually contributing to poor health. Sometimes, one of the other two linkages will lead you to awareness of the big picture.

To truly improve your health, you must look at your outer circle. Examine each aspect, and carry out an assessment to see which elements could be detracting from your health. Honestly evaluate your personal outlook, confidence, stress level, entertainment choices, relationships, career, finances, spirituality, physical environment, and frequency of exercise. If any of these areas are drastically out of balance, they could be detracting from your health. Once you become aware of these things, you can move on to other linkages.

Likewise, you must perform an accurate assessment of your eating habits. It is now normal to eat out rather than have a home-cooked meal. When we eat out, we are bombarded with large portions containing little to no nutrition. This is one fact that everyone should be aware of. These types of eating habits are negatively contributing to our society's health. By changing your habits and the actual foods you eat, you will become aware of the negative impact they could have on your health.

Once you are aware of something that is detracting from your vitality, you must have the knowledge to work on that area. You can obtain the necessary information through many avenues. In some cases, you will need to see a doctor, coach, boss, relative, or spiritual leader to obtain the necessary guidance to help you deal with an unhealthy habit or relationship. In other cases, you can obtain the knowledge through research, books, or the Internet. Finally, you may have to do some experimentation on your own to obtain knowledge that will truly enhance your health.

You must also come up with a manageable plan of attack. Some changes, like quitting smoking, will take considerable work. You might have to try several different approaches, and take baby steps. Creating small, manageable sub-goals will make a daunting task less so. Try not to become overwhelmed, and don't be too hard on yourself if you happen to slip up once in a while. The key is to continually make strides in the right direction.

Motivation may well represent the toughest aspect of the linkages. You can have a great deal of knowledge and awareness about something that is causing you to have less-than-optimal health, but you cannot effect real change until you have the motivation. Often, the mere desire to change does not provide the necessary discipline to actually make the difference. Try to find alternative motivation. Also, I do not suggest using your external self-image (your looks) as your only source of motivation. This will improve on its own, as you improve your health.

My motivation is to be an example for other people, but most importantly, to stand as an example to my kids. I want to be able to play in the park with my great-grandchildren, not sit in my wheelchair in a nursing home.

An endless number of things can motivate you to be healthier. Your motivation might stem from a positive event, like a wedding; or a negative occurrence, like a health scare. You could be motivated by a loved one's health issue or death. These events can be very emotional, but you still have to gain the necessary education, and make a plan with sub-goals, in order to be successful.

6
DATING

To me, my wife Jadelle looked particularly beautiful when we were dating, on our wedding day, when we had our children, and when I returned from deployments. This is not to say that I don't think she is beautiful all the time; but I can distinctly remember thinking "wow" at each of these particular times in our lives, when we really had the time to appreciate one other. I therefore want to start this chapter off with some advice. One of the biggest mistakes we can all fall into in our relationships is taking our significant other for granted. Appreciate your loved one *all* the time, both in action and in words. This will start you off on the track to a healthy relationship.

Most of us can probably remember the first time we started dating "the one." We could not think of anything else, and were continually counting down the minutes until we would see each other again. As time goes on, however, we have to find ways to balance the rest of our lives with our relationship. Balance is the most difficult skill to master. You will quickly find out when you are out of balance, because you will slip up in some areas in your life. From the beginning of your relationship, you will both have to figure out how to balance your connection with the other demands of your life.

As your relationship develops, remember to find ways to communicate effectively. Communication is the key to relationships, but many people do not pay much attention to good/deep communication in the beginning. It is imperative to find ways to express your point of view so the other person can understand you. You also have to make a concerted effort to listen to what the other person is saying. Sometimes, what you actually mean is not always communicated correctly. Take the time to be clear about your desires and ensure that you understand your significant other's. Do not assume anything. Sometimes it is the delivery of what you are saying that is most important, so think about how you say things. This may sound simplistic, but lack of communication can cause significant problems later on in a relationship.

Compromise can be practiced along the same lines. The more you communicate, the more you may find times that you do not agree. It is healthy to disagree, but it is not healthy to let it linger and pull at you. It is best to talk things out, and make compromises that will better your relationship in the long run. It may even be necessary to agree to disagree; just make sure that there are no strings attached to the outcome. You should always be able to express your love, and put disagreements behind you. It is a good practice to either put a time limit on bringing up the past, or decide to learn from past issues and then forget them in the sense that you do not continue to bring them up at every opportunity.

At this time in your life together, keep health always in the back of your mind. As you start deciding upon activities to do together, try to involve the healthiest possible choices. You may wish to exercise strenuously together, or simply take a walk, giving you time to talk and reflect. Cooking together starts you off with a healthy, collaborative way of providing nutrition to your bodies.

7
NEWLYWEDS, THINKING ABOUT CHILDREN, AND PRENATAL HEALTH

Although this chapter is written from the perspective of a male and female with the desire to conceive children naturally, all of the recommendations given will inevitably contribute to any type of relationship or adoption situation.

First and foremost, from the time you decide to get married, get into the habit of having regular discussions about your future. Talk about what you want your married life to look like in one, five, and ten years. These discussions should include things like schooling, careers, finances, and family. I know it may not always seem practical, but you will be better-prepared when you plan for major life events.

One of the most important things you can plan for is the long-term health of your family. It should come as no surprise that I recommend starting out your relationship by choosing healthy activities and good nutrition. From your first days together, try to adjust your lifestyle to take advantage of the recommendations listed in the earlier chapters of this book.

If children are in your future, it is never too early to start eating for fertility and prenatal health. Studies have shown that there exists a positive relationship between a healthy pre-conception diet and healthy childbirth. The challenge is *getting* to that healthy pre-conception diet. Studies have shown that most women, especially in the reproductive age, have diets that lack calcium, iron, vitamins A, C, B6, E, folic acid, zinc, and magnesium.

The first, immediate area to focus upon should be any known habits or food choices that contribute to poor health. Some habits, such as cigarette use, are non-negotiable. There is too much evidence showing that smoking is detrimental to your health and cannot possibly start a baby off well, either. Another habit would be drug use. It may be obvious that illicit drug use is not good for your health, but if you are continually taking even prescription drugs, you should talk to your doctor about reassessing your true need for them. Often, you can make adjustments to your diet, or take more natural supplements to treat a chronic ailment.

I feel very strongly about artificial sweeteners and colors, as well, which have no positive benefits. I believe they can actually be harmful to you and very dangerous to fetal development, so you should try to start weaning off of them before getting pregnant, then stay away from them altogether. Finally, there are a few things that you should probably try to limit during pre-conception (and stay away from during pregnancy), like alcohol and caffeine. There is currently a lot of controversy about caffeine, but when it comes right down to it, your body does not need it. Caffeine is a powerful stimulant, and you do not want this during fetal development.

I would recommend taking a pre-natal multivitamin to ensure that you are getting adequate nutrients, but you should be getting most of what you need from a healthy diet rich in the foods listed below. After each category, you'll see a suggested dosage range, as recommended by the American Pregnancy Association. The doses will either be in micrograms per day (mcg/d) or milligrams per day (mg/d).

The following dietary recommendations are good for both men and women during pre-conception. They will be pretty similar to those you read about in previous chapters, but this time, I will discuss why they are important during this particular time in your relationship. Always consult your physician before making any dietary changes. As always, a diet low in processed foods and added sugars, made up of mostly fruits, vegetables, whole grains, lean meat, and dairy, will be best for both of you. Your beverage of choice should be water.

Folic acid has gotten the most attention in the last few years due to its protection of the developing fetus. Research has shown that it is crucial to DNA replication and cell division. It has also been linked to the prevention of spinal defects. You can find folic acid in green leafy vegetables, legumes, citrus fruits, breads, and cereals enriched with folate (400-1000 mcg/d).

Vitamin A is important for vision, fetal growth, immunity, and skin repair. Lack of vitamin A has been linked to birth defects related to the cardiovascular system, cranial development, and development of the thymus. Sources of vitamin A are leafy green vegetables, eggs, dairy, and carrots (700-3000 mcg/d).

Vitamin D assists your body's ability to properly use calcium and phosphorous. This is very important in bone formation and for the immune system. Your body can produce vitamin D from exposure to the sun (just be sure not to get a sunburn.) Sources of vitamin D include milk, fish, orange juice, cereals, eggs, and cheese (5-50 mcg/d).

Calcium is essential for bone formation and bodily maintenance. It is crucial to the development of the fetal skeletal system. Sources of calcium include milk, dairy, green leafy vegetables, chia and flax seeds, nuts, tofu, and dried herbs (1300-2500 mg/d).

Iron is the most common deficiency worldwide, and lack of it can cause anemia during pregnancy. Low iron can lead to insufficient amounts of oxygen getting to the developing fetus. Low iron (and therefore low oxygen levels) during pregnancy can lead to lower birth weight and possible developmental brain issues such as learning disabilities. Iron is mostly found in lean meat and poultry (15-45 mg/d).

Iodine deficiency is the single most preventable cause of brain damage. Iodine is important for proper thyroid function, as well. It has been added to most table salts, but I would suggest sea salt. Iodine is also in seaweed, shrimp, navy beans, the peel of baked potato, and milk (150 mcg/d).

Zinc is important for the production and repair of DNA. This is especially crucial for the developing fetus. Foods high in zinc include shellfish, poultry, beans, nuts, whole grains, and dairy products (8-40 mg/d).

Essential Fatty Acids (EFA) such as *linoleic*, *alpha-linoleic*, *arachidonic*, and *docosahexaenoic* acids (DHA) are crucial for cell membrane structure, central nervous system development, and the brain. Our bodies cannot synthesize these, so we must get them from our diet. These are the "good fats," and are also known as *omegas*. The best source of these fats is fish, but you can also get them from nuts, chia seeds, and "good" oils such as olive oil. A fish oil supplement can also help (at least 1000 mg/d).

If you keep these key substances in mind, you will inevitably get all of the other important vitamins and minerals that I have not mentioned here. As far as shopping for these items, I think it is important to try to buy all foods in the least-processed state possible. Non-GMO and organic foods are better, as are local foods. All three usually limit the amount of pesticides, insecticides, and artificial fertilizers used.

Don't forget your outer circle throughout this time. Building a strong relationship with your spouse is of the utmost importance. Communicate, communicate, communicate. Evaluate the people that you interact with on a daily basis. Look at the environments that you find yourself in. Your habits and environment are crucial right now. You should ensure that the environment you put yourself in is not hurting or detracting in any way from your healthy body. Strive to maintain a balance in your day to day life. Make every effort to maintain a good exercise regimen at all times.

8

DURING PREGNANCY

This is probably the most important stage of your life together. By following the suggestions in the previous chapter, you and your spouse will have prepared your bodies for pregnancy. Since your physical self is inevitably going to be stressed during this period, you will have to make a concerted effort to eat as suggested in the previous chapter, and to ensure that you are getting proper nutrition not only for you, but for your developing child.

As far as eating and weight gain during pregnancy, it is important to eat often, so you do not feel hungry. It is crucial to maintain a healthy weight during pregnancy. You will obviously gain weight, but too much or too little can put you and your fetus at risk. A body that is greatly underweight or overweight stresses your internal systems. If internal systems are stressed, they will be unable to properly dedicate resources to the developing baby.

Now, a little about fetal development. It is important to understand each phase of the development of your fetus as your pregnancy goes on. This will help you ensure that you are staying healthy. Many developmental disorders have been traced to specific times during pregnancy, and can usually be attributed to a nutritional deficiency.

The following represent the general time frames for development. Each person is a little different, so keep this in mind while reading the timeline.

The embryo stage starts 6 to 12 days after conception; this is when the blastocyst (group of cells) is embedded in the uterine lining. By week three, the fetus is developing its brain, spinal cord, heart and gastrointestinal tract. This is very important to realize; some people do not even know that they are pregnant at this time. This is why it is never too early to start living a healthy.

During weeks four and five, the arms and legs are starting to form. The baby's heart is beating, and blood is flowing through its body. Remember, everything that goes into your developing baby comes from you. At this point, the physical areas are starting to develop where the eyes and ears will later be.

Week six starts the development of lungs, jaws, and nose. The hands and feet are starting to form fingers and toes. By the end of week seven, all of the body's organs are developing. Hair starts growing, and the eyelids and tongue begin to form.

In week eight, the ears are continuing to develop, both internally and externally. Bones are now forming, and muscles can contract. Although the baby is only one inch long, it is now forming facial features.

During weeks nine to thirteen, the fetus will grow to three inches in length. Although the genitals have formed, they are still not visible via ultrasound. The fetus can now make fists, and its head is half the size of the body. This is the end of the first trimester, and as you can see, quite a bit of development has occurred thus far.

The second trimester starts with week 14 to 16. The baby's skin is transparent, and the baby starts swallowing and defecating (producing meconium). The organs are stepping up their own functioning, and the mother may start to feel the baby move. By the end of this period, the baby is about six inches long and weighs about four ounces.

Weeks 17 through 20 lead to quite a bit of movement felt by the mother. The eyebrows, eyelashes, and fingernails are now growing. The fetal heartbeat can be heard via stethoscope. Also, the vernix (a white pasty substance) is forming on the skin to protect it from the amniotic fluid.

During weeks 21 to 23, the baby's skin is becoming less transparent. The liver and pancreas are working very hard to keep up with development. The baby is now 10 to 11 inches long, and weighs over one pound.

Weeks 24 to 26 round out the second trimester. By the end of this time period, the baby could survive on its own with tremendous medical support. The baby has developed sleeping and waking cycles, has a startle reflex, and has developed lung air sacs. The brain has really started developing, and the nervous system is functioning. By the end of this trimester, the baby is about 14 inches long and weighs over two pounds.

The third trimester starts with weeks 27 to 32. At this point, the bones are formed, but still pliable. The eyelids are now opening. During weeks 33 to 36, the baby starts to get situated in a head-down position in preparation for delivery. The baby is gaining weight rapidly, and is now about 16-19 inches long.

The last month of the trimester is when the mother is providing her little one with antibodies against disease. The baby is moving around a lot less, because it is taking up most of the available space. All organs are functioning, and development is nearing completion. The baby is considered full-term at 38 weeks, and will usually be born measuring between 19 to 21 inches long and weighing between six and ten pounds.

By this point, you have a good understanding of fetal development and the essential elements to nutrition. A discussion before the big day arrives should cover what you want your delivery process to look like. Things to consider include: natural vs. medicated, and vaginal vs. C-section. Who do you want to be present, and who might be able to help you? Some of these consider-ations may be outside of your control, but you should make sure that your desires are known to each other and to the hospital staff. I would recommend trying to do as much as you can naturally.

During your entire pregnancy, you will be working on your outer circle as much as your inner circle in all of the choices you make. Assess the support circle that will help you during pregnancy and after the baby is born. Don't forget to continually reassess your one, five, and ten-year goals—now with a child in mind. Throughout this time, you should start preparing for the baby's arrival. This is another time that communication will be very important. You can also begin to establish routines and duties in your relationship for after the baby is born. Surround yourself with people that can support you through these changes in your life.

9
BIRTH AND THE FIRST FEW YEARS

The day has finally arrived! You should have a very good idea of how you want things to go—and hopefully, they will go as planned. Natural childbirth is the best option, if it is possible for you. Research suggests that this process is helpful for developing a healthy immune system for the baby. Always be prepared for the unexpected, however, and retain your ability to go with the flow and make informed decisions as the process unfolds.

Ensure that you take advantage of the time you have at the hospital in order to receive advice from the medical staff. Ask as many questions as you can, and listen to their advice. You will certainly receive information and instruction about breastfeeding. Although the baby's nutrition starts at conception, breastfeeding is the most important introduction to nourishment outside of the womb.

Breast milk is best for your baby, and its benefits extend well beyond basic nutrition. In addition to providing all of the vitamins and nutrients your baby needs in the first six months of life, breast milk is also packed with disease-fighting substances that protect your little one from illness.

If, for some reason, you cannot breastfeed, be very careful about the formula you choose. Many of the big-name brands still do not provide babies with what they need; and worse, they can be packed with genetically modified soy. In many cases, they are also loaded with unnecessary sugar, so do your research to make the best decision for your little one. Look for organic or non-GMO brands.

After you have brought your new baby home, figure out how you are going to split up duties and responsibilities so that you can both still function. It will be important to continue paying careful attention to your nutrition and exercise (within doctor's guidance). Proper nutrition is important for producing breast milk for the baby, and for keeping you both functioning optimally. Incorporating exercise in the form of walks will get you into a good routine that you can easily continue.

The baby will probably seem to be eating and sleeping almost all the time! Because of their small stomachs, babies eat approximately every two hours. They also require adequate sleep in order to grow. Remember, your baby is training you as much as you are teaching him or her. Stick to the routines that work for all of you, and remain aware that everything you do has an effect on the baby.

It's okay not to pick them up every single time they whimper. Even at this young age, babies should learn to self-comfort a bit and figure things out for them-selves—within reason. Babies often need only three simple things: to be breastfed (or fed), have their diaper changed, and/or to be helped along with a burp. If you've checked all of these needs and your baby is still fussy, examine the mother's diet to rule out gassiness for the baby. Commonly, vegetables from the *brassica* family, when eaten by the breastfeeding mother, can cause colic or discomfort in the baby's digestion. These foods include broccoli, cabbage, cauliflower, and Brussels sprouts.

The following feeding suggestions are gathered from a conglomeration of information sources; all of them should be discussed with your doctor.

Since your baby's digestive system is still developing, they should only have breast milk or formula (if necessary) for the first four months. For the first few days of breastfeeding, your baby will only be getting colostrum, which is thick and very valuable to permanent immune health. When your baby is a newborn, he or she will probably have only two wet diapers per day. A little later, after the mother's milk comes in, they will have somewhere between five and eight wet diapers per day. Runny bowel movements in the first month occur two to three times daily, and become less frequent after that.

It is normal for baby to initially lose a little weight immediately after leaving the hospital. A good rule of thumb for growth is five to ten ounces per week for the first month. In months two and three, they should gain five to eight ounces per week. In months three to six, they should gain between two and five ounces a week; and from six to twelve months, they should gain one to two ounces per week.

Somewhere between four and six months of age is when you can start to introduce other (solid) foods. Some signs that your baby is ready include the ability to hold their head up, sit well in a highchair, make a chewing motion, demonstrate steady weight gain as described above, show interest in food, close their mouth around a spoon, and move their tongue around. Your baby may not do all of these, but they are all indications that he or she is getting ready for solid food. You should consult your doctor, as well.

On the subject of the best types of foods to choose, you could start with an iron-fortified cereal or pureed fruits and vegetables. I strongly encourage trying to make your own pureed food if you can; this way, you'll know exactly what is in it. Ensure that you strain the pureed food so that no chunks are missed. Small, easy-to-use food mills, widely available for online purchase, allow you to safely and easily puree foods for your little one. Introduce your baby to the foods you eat and have in your house. I also encourage you to try to get the widest possible variety of fruits and vegetables as time goes on. I believe this will lead children to be less picky eaters as they grow up. As far as cereal goes, there is plenty of time for that, so don't *just* use cereal; try out many things, in moderation.

As far as portion size goes, you should start with a teaspoon a day. The consistency should be very runny, and you can mix breast milk with it to make it runnier, if necessary. You can increase to one tablespoon twice a day as you see that your baby is taking food well. Over time, you can make the consistency a little thicker.

From six to eight months, you can continue to increase the variety of foods you are introducing. You can also start including pureed (and strained) meats, organic tofu, and legumes. Just ensure that you cook items such as carrots and beans well before pureeing. At this point, you can give your baby three to nine tablespoons of cereals a day in addition to breast milk over two to three meals. You can vary the type of cereal a little, too (oats, barley, rice, or wheat). Try one teaspoon of fruit, and gradually increase the amount to ¼ cup to ½ cup over two to three meals. Use the same guidelines for vegetables. For meats and legumes, you can supplement them at each meal, and if necessary, reduce the amount of cereal to get these items in. It is recommended that you introduce new foods one at a time, and wait two or three days before introducing another. During this time, you will be able to notice if your baby seems to be allergic to any new items.

Somewhere between eight and ten months of age is when you should begin noticing that your baby can start picking things up with their thumb and forefinger. Also, babies can transfer items from one hand to another, and make chewing motions with their mouths. These are signs that you can probably start introducing more solid foods.

The foods you should start out with should be mashed-up fruits and vegetables. You can also use small amounts of other foods, like eggs and cheese. The majority of these soft foods should be fruits and cooked vegetables, followed by protein and dairy. There are many products sold that cater to this age. I would simply caution you to check the ingredients and ensure that your child is eating the most pure and unprocessed foods available. I believe that taking a few extra minutes to prepare foods for your child will enhance their health far more than just buying convenient packaged foods.

From this point on, slowly increase the foods listed above, and introduce new foods as your baby can handle them. After twelve months, you can add cow's milk, and continue to try new things. Always be conscious of which foods agree with your child and which ones do not. Also, keep an open mind, and don't force anything that doesn't seem to be working. When looking for new foods, try to stay away from items with loads of sugar, artificial colors, and additives.

Somewhere between 24 and 36 months, your child will probably want to try to feed themselves. Encourage this, and assist them. They may also want to make food choices. This is fine, but try to still make sure that they are getting a variety of foods, and eating plenty of vegetables and fruit. Children cannot eat too much of these, and this will contribute to their overall health. Your child should be getting a variety of fiber sources, vitamins, and nutrients from "good" foods. Even though this can be tough when you're not in your home environment, always try to ensure you are making the best food choices while at a restaurant or in other people's homes. Do not hesitate to ask for better choices, even if they are not available on the menu or at a party.

Always consult your doctor when making major changes to your child's diet, and start from the earliest months with a variety of healthy and unprocessed foods. This will give your child a very healthy start that should continue to provide them with benefits throughout their life.

At this age, children are not too young to pay attention to their outer circle. They are learning who they can trust. They are also constantly learning from their environment. In my opinion, the most important thing to show your child is love, but that does not mean you should always give in to them. It's up to you to establish reasonable, healthy boundaries and rules. It is never too early to explain consequences of your child's actions. I am not a fan of baby talk or assuming that children do not understand. They might not understand in the way you and I do, but they do understand.

Do not neglect your outer circle either. Communication with your spouse is very important during this period as well. You both have to be on the same sheet of music with each other's feelings and desires. You will need ways to relieve stress from the baby and the changes in your life. Exercise is always a good way to deal with stress. Do not underestimate the need for good relationships with friends and family members. These relationships should help you manage stress, give you an outlet, and even some advice during trying times.

10
SCHOOL-AGED YEARS

In the United States, children start daycare and pre-school at an early age. Some parents operate on blind trust that schools will automatically do what is best for their child. I am not saying that these institutions would intentionally try to endanger your child's health and well-being—just that you, as the parents, are the only ones who know what is truly best for your child. It is your responsibility to ensure that the places that you take your child are aligned with your beliefs. I also recommend packing your child's foods, so that you know for sure that your child is eating is what is best for them. This takes a little extra time and planning, but you will know that you have done all you can to provide for them in the best possible way.

The key here is ensuring that your child has a well-rounded diet. There are always going to be children who only want to eat chicken fingers and macaroni and cheese. With all children, it is never too early to explain the benefits of eating healthfully. It helps to make preparing foods fun. Mix flavors, have your child assist in preparation, and make the meal look appealing. You can have a lot of fun making your child's food look fun to eat—by making a face out of pieces of sliced fruit, for example. These little touches can make a big difference.

Remember that you should never allow your child to say, "I don't like that." Encourage them to try something several times, prepared in different ways. Remember, all food does not have to taste like dessert to be good. After trying a food several times, children will usually get used to it, especially if you are setting a good example by eating right, too. As a last resort, there are plenty of ways to "hide" nutritious foods in a meal. There are a few cookbooks out there that could help, as well.

Most children get too much sugar in the beverages they drink. Water should be their primary source of hydration. Milk is fine, but you should try to ensure that it is organic, or at the very least, that it does not contain growth hormones. Juices should stay to a minimum, perhaps one cup a day or so. When you take the juice from the fruit, you miss its most valuable part, which is the fiber. When you eat a whole fruit, the fiber slows its digestion so your body can deal with the accompanying sugars. When you drink juice, on the other hand, you dump a bunch of sugar in your body without the fiber to help in processing. This allows more of it to throw your insulin levels into imbalance, leading to sugar highs and lows. As a result, more gets stored as fat. Teas without sugar, especially tasty herbal blends, are a great alternative or compromise. Obviously, there can be caffeine in teas, so you have to drink these in moderation or choose an herbal tea that is naturally caffeine free; but you could mix a little fruit juice with unsweetened tea to make a delicious beverage.

At this point, it is really important to ensure that when you shop, you are reading the labels. Many parents buy (and children want to eat) packaged foods. Some packaged foods are alright, but you should try to limit them. If you do buy packaged foods, ensure that you select foods that are low in sugar and saturated fats, with no artificial sweeteners, GMOs, or artificial colors.

You should always have healthy snack options available. Children are constantly burning calories, so they will naturally be hungry more often than adults. The key to healthy snacks is to select foods low in sugar and high in fiber. The best choices are vegetables or fruits, but nuts and non-microwaveable popcorn are also very good options.

With that said, you should not transform eating into a chore, or completely deprive children of "treats." When shopping for treats, simply compare labels. I have found that if you are looking for cookies, for example, you can buy a brand with 25 g of sugar per serving, or a brand with just 10 g of sugar. They are both cookies, but one would be a little healthier than the other. One way to ensure that you don't go overboard is to avoid keeping these foods in your house as constantly-available choices. It is more of a treat to go out to the ice cream shop than to just get ice cream out of the freezer whenever you want it.

Eating out is another area in which a bit of caution will serve you well. I am by no means saying you shouldn't eat out at all—but you should definitely try to make good decisions about where to eat and what to order for your children. In most areas, there are restaurants opening now that specialize in healthier options, and I would suggest those first, so you can make better choices. Be very careful with children's menus. Most restaurants have very unhealthy children's menus, because they think that is what children want. Don't be afraid to share your meal with your child, or order some side dishes of healthier foods. Finally, do not hesitate to ask the server to substitute a healthier option like vegetables instead of French fries.

As children get a bit older, they learn quite a bit about their outer circle. They are experiencing many new environments such as play groups, school, and sports/activities. It is important to always check in about what happened each day, and if they mention a behavior they saw that you do not approve of, explain that this is not acceptable, and that they should not do it. Always reinforce respect and discipline. Oftentimes, teachers and coaches do not have enough time to teach these principles, because they are constantly dealing with the children who need the most attention (whether positive or negative).

As time goes on in school, it becomes important to teach children not only how to interact with others, but also how to comfort themselves. I have already mentioned the importance of discipline and respect, but children often do not get enough guidance in how to manage their time. This will help them as they get more homework and participate in a greater variety of activities. Always reinforce the importance of being loving, caring, and a life-long learner. When children ask questions (and I know they will), try to give them accurate answers. Encourage them to do research on their own. When they are young, they will be learning how to read and use a computer. Teach them how to find out information for themselves, and encourage them to share what they have learned with you. You can also encourage little science experiments, if you have the time. I really think it is important not to simply tell them all of the answers; children will learn a lot more, and retain what they have learned, if they are allowed to figure things out on their own.

Again, do not neglect yourself or your spouse through this period of your life.

11
TEENAGE YEARS

Our children are bombarded by hundreds of media ads each day, and it can be challenging for them to make the correct nutritional choices. Hopefully, by this time in your child's life, they will understand for themselves the benefits of healthy choices, and proper self-care will not seem like a chore. Many of the children your kids go to school with will display the results of poor nutrition, both physically and mentally. If you have been explaining nutritional principles throughout their lives, this will not come as a surprise. Hopefully, your children will act as ambassadors for healthy choices rather than outcasts.

You have probably tried, by this time, to ingrain in your children that mealtime is a pleasant time when the family gathers. They should feel comfortable with the amount of food they eat, not forced to eat more or less. Food should not symbolize a reward or a substitute for comfort. Everyone in the family eats healthy food. The refrigerator is stocked with healthy foods. Everyone can help prepare healthy food; it is not just one person's responsibility. Mealtime is a time to talk with other family members, and share about the day.

Teens will start to consume more calories than ever before. They are really growing at this point in their lives, and quickly developing into young adults. In fact, they will gain 20 percent of their height and 50 percent of their weight during puberty. Adequate nutrition will ensure that their bodies develop properly, and will keep them healthy as their physical selves work so hard to develop. Particular nutritional areas to be mindful of include protein, calcium, iron, folate, and zinc.

Although all macro- and micronutrients are important for development, the items listed above seem to be ones that teens commonly do not get enough of. Teenagers need 45 to 60 g of protein each day, and they can get it by eating lean meat, nuts, legumes, dairy, and certain vegetables. Teens should get about 1200 mg of calcium per day to build strong bones as they grow. They can get this through calcium-fortified foods and green leafy vegetables. Soda and sugary foods fight against strong bones by leaching calcium from the skeletal structure, so they should be kept to a minimum (and hopefully, by this time, that is the norm in your children's lives, anyway).

Teens need about 12 to 15 mg of iron a day. Iron helps the blood carry oxygen to the muscles and the brain, and also builds the immune system. This is particularly important for girls because of their menstrual cycle. Iron is found in lean meat, leafy greens, beans, nuts, and whole grains. Teens also need about 400 mcg of folate each day. This is necessary for cell growth and development, DNA production, and creation of red blood cells. A diet rich in fruits, vegetables, beans, and lean meat can provide adequate folate. Zinc is need-ed for the reproductive, endocrine, neurological, and immune systems. It also prevents DNA damage, and teenagers should have between 9 and 11 mg of it each day. Good sources of zinc include lean meats, dairy, beans, nuts, and mushrooms.

Proper nutrition will also keep teenagers' skin clear, and help them to sleep better, think clearly, and perform optimally in activities. Although their lives are very busy, you can still ensure that they have ways to obtain healthy foods. Good breakfasts and snacks will help immeasurably in this area. Be sure that your children have access to a healthy meal for lunch, whether they bring their own food or purchase it.

Although nutrition is very important for keeping a teenager's inner circle balanced, at this point in their lives, they may also need some assistance in the outer circle area. As we all know, a lot of things go on at school that have nothing to do with academic learning. This is not always a bad thing, but your children may need some support in handling these issues. As discussed earlier, balancing relationships, work, school, and environment can be very challenging.

My best advice is to be there to listen, without jumping to judge or fix situations. You are teaching your child how to react to situations they have never encountered before, but will have to encounter for the rest of their lives.

Teens have to figure out how to reason through the pros and cons of any given decision, and must learn to deal with the consequences. This is one area in which the adult brain differs from the teen brain. Teenagers are still trying to define boundaries for themselves. This is why they may seem impulsive at times. They are developing the part of their brains associated with risk-taking and reward, and coming to a broader understanding of how the world works. Up to this point, children take in all of the information they can, and rely on parents to help them sort out what is important. As teens, they now start figuring out what's important for themselves, and this is why they seem not to want to listen to parents anymore.

My best advice is try to be patient. Realize that your teenager still needs your example and guidance, even if they do not seem to want it. It is your job to adjust the delivery, so they can hear your message and receive it.

One more thing to think about is your teenager's future. The things they do—or don't do—at this age will effectively open or close doors for them in the future. Remember that their grades and activities are what they will use to get into college or as material for their resume. They should take advantage of every opportunity they can to set themselves apart from the average kid without being obsessive.

Don't forget about balance in your life.

12
SELF-SUFFICENCY

The teenage years mark the time when your children are planning to graduate from high school and go off to college. I do not believe college is for everyone, especially for a child who has had a hard time and dislikes school. I think they should do something that makes them happy, but that can also pay the bills. There is a career out there for everyone, though usually some sort of training is required. It is important to get that training. There is nothing wrong with technical careers, such as plumber or electrician; but your kids should have some sort of plan, and keep goals in mind for their adult lives. As you may have guessed from my bio, I am a fan of joining the military, especially for someone who does not know what they want to do with themselves right out of high school. This gives them adequate time to mature; a strong sense of discipline, teamwork, and respect; a world view; experience; and leadership skills, all of which remain extremely valuable even if the person does not want to stay in the military.

As you can guess, the outer circle is where older teenagers will be focusing quite a lot of their energy. It is your job to support their decision-making process as they figure out what they want to do after high school. As mentioned above, if they want to do something other than college, support them; but help them figure out the best path to success for them personally. This may require that you do some research or talk to people in a field with which you are unfamiliar, but you can give the best advice if you are well-informed. Don't get too upset when teens don't always take your advice right away. They have to make these decisions for themselves, and your role is to try to support them however you can.

In terms of college, we have to do a lot of research as parents, too. College is much more complicated than it used to be. The application process is different. Make sure you understand it with your children, and help them plan ahead to fill out applications. You'll need to help them figure out where to apply. These days, colleges are often more specialized in certain disciplines.

It helps your children for the future if you can figure out which colleges are the best for your child's area of interest. Help your teenager figure out their chances of getting into these colleges—not only grade-wise, but tuition-wise, as well.

Once you have narrowed down the schools your child is most interested in, make plans to visit them. Be cautious of all the "advertising" a school will do. On the campus tour, they will show all of the great conveniences your student will have access to; but your kids are there first and foremost for the education, so make sure the college offers what will truly suit your child. When it comes right down to it, they have to make the best decision for them without worrying about other things, like who else might be going there.

Even if you do not get grey hair simply from going through this process, know that it will feel even more difficult when your child is preparing to actually leave—and when they are gone. Your teenager should have a firm understanding of how to manage money and how to deal with other people. Time management will have to be learned very quickly. You will have to gauge how much help they will need to move along in this part of their life. No matter how much your child needs, be sure they know that you are there to support them, listen, and offer advice. You may have to remind them of their goals and priorities from time to time, but now is the time to sit back and just be there, whenever you are needed.

Other aspects of the outer circle older teenagers will have to deal with at this time include career, relationships, friends and lovers, and environment. In terms of career, they may want to complete internships or gain work experience, either during the academic year or over the summer. This provides great material and substance for their resume, and will set them up for success after college.

As far as relationships go, just be aware that both friendships and love relationships are happening. Hopefully, your teenager will choose friends who truly look out for them and do not participate in too many crazy habits. My best advice on love is to prolong it until after schooling. Obviously, you cannot dictate this; but it is time for them to really prepare themselves for the future. Your child's studies should be priority one, and if they do find the perfect person, their significant other will understand, too, and respect their wishes.

Environment can offer the most enhancing or detracting elements during the college years. Clubs, academic work, internships, and activities can really make for a fulfilling time at university, but the party environment, and all that goes along with it, can play a significantly distracting role. Relieving stress through exercise is a much better choice. Older teenagers will have to figure out how to balance everything, and hopefully, they will realize that they do not have much time for partying.

As far as the inner circle goes, college students must remember to get proper amounts of sleep. In college, it usually seems like there is not enough time to do everything that is necessary, but this is where time management comes in. Sleep is very important to keep the immune system up and the brain sharp. Students should plan for it, just like everything else they need to do each day.

Your child should, by now, have a firm grasp of the importance of nutrition, but you may have to help them get creative about balancing this with everything else they have going on. Reminding them to cook once and eat twice (or more) helps. Also, healthy snack choices are important on-the-go and in between classes. College students have to continue to make the best possible choices, wherever they end up eating: in a dining hall on campus, at a restaurant, or in their dorm/apartment. Adequate (or even optimal) nutrition will allow them to deal with all of the stresses of college life and keep them healthy, as well—perfectly able to learn and retain crucial information for their future careers.

Your health is still important during this period.

13
EMPTY NEST YEARS

The empty-nest years represent a time for you and your spouse to reconnect with each other. You'll have the chance to really focus on your outer circle. During the time when you are raising children, they are the focus of your energy, as they should be. Raising children is the toughest job in the world, especially if you care enough to do it in the best way you possibly can. There were probably plenty of times in the last two decades when you split your time, effort and energy so your child could receive the attention they needed, at the expense of attention to your spouse. This is not to say that you should not have tried to balance your efforts to ensure your spouse felt your love, as well—but I do recognize the difficulty.

In the area of your outer circle, now is the time to make special efforts to reconnect with your spouse. Some suggestions might be special lunches or dinners, which were not so common or frequent when the children were growing up. Go out to movies, and look for events to attend that you both enjoy. Surprise each other. Do activities that you have never done before.

You can also consider your environment, and how to make things a little easier on both of you. When you are downsizing your space or responsibilities, this may, in fact, give you more time to reconnect. Go for walks together. Make sure you take the time to listen to each other and enjoy one another's company.

You will both have to figure out how to remain a positive influence, or at least a listening ear, for your child who has now moved out of the house. This can be one of the most difficult things to adjust to. You have to realize that your children now have their own lives and make their own decisions, but you must still be available to help when needed. This is a time to cultivate your listening skills, and help them to recognize the pros, cons, and long-term repercussions of their choices.

Perhaps the most difficult thing we wrestle with at this time is the amount of support (especially financial support) that we continue to give our children. On the one hand, you want to help them out however you can; on the other, you do not want to make them dependent upon you. This could drain the savings you've been stockpiling to use when you retire, causing you to take on unnecessary debt. A right or wrong answer here does not exist, because every situation is different; just be conscious of what you are doing and the repercussions of your actions. At some point, grown children have to fend for themselves, and it is perfectly alright to let them fail, if that is what they need to do to in order to truly learn from their decisions. Remember, our lives are the result of the decisions we make. You can try to guide your children, but they will ultimately have to live with their own choices.

As far as personal care goes, continue to incorporate exercise into your life. Weight training can be important for building or at least maintaining muscle. As we get older, we slowly lose muscle, so if you never try to replenish it, this will be more difficult to get around when you are older. Remember that exercise is the way you keep your body's systems performing well. It will allow you to live a long, pain-free, disease-free life. As a bonus, it's an excellent way to manage stress. Don't hesitate to go out for walks together.

What about your inner circle? If you haven't noticed by this time, our bodies change as we get older, so nutrition becomes absolutely crucial to your well-being. Hopefully, you have been eating well this whole time, so you will not see the "signs" of aging as much. One common misconception about the diseases common to older people is that they just pop up, all of a sudden, when you reach a certain age. This could not be further from the truth. In reality, you may have been beating up your body your whole life, and it could finally be giving in a little as you age, manifesting neglect or chronic abuse as disease. It is never too late to get your nutrition on track.

The good news is that there is nothing you have to do much differently, as long as you have been following what I have discussed thus far in this book. Here are the essential areas to pay attention to.

Eat a variety of foods. Pay particular attention to eating as many fruits and vegetables as you can. Choose whole grains whenever possible. Include essential fatty acids, or good fats, in your diet. Keep the amount of trans-fats and saturated fats to a minimum. Try to increase your calcium intake with green leafy vegetables, nuts, fish, and seeds. Choose foods low in salt; it is implicated in many of the "older person" diseases.

Limit your alcohol consumption. Finally, if you see yourself putting on extra weight, take a look at your diet and see if there is anything you can do to prevent or mitigate this.

14
GRANDPARENT YEARS

These are the years during which you are supposed to
spoil your grandchildren. In order to be healthy enough
to keep up with them, hopefully you have been balancing your health, as I have suggested. As you get
older, you lose muscle each year, so it is crucially important to keep exercising. This will slow down muscle
loss and keep your body's systems in working order. As
always, eating well will keep you feeling healthy in the
optimal sense.

You will have to realize that many things have changed
since you were raising children. There is a very difficult and delicate balance between giving advice and
respecting your child's way of parenting. My best sug-
gestion is to do more listening and offer advice when

requested, but do not insist or get upset if your grown children do not take your advice.

One of the biggest challenges you will experience will be in balancing your outer circle at this stage in your life. If you are still working and/or active in your community, you have those obligations; but now you also have the desire to spend time with your grandchildren, as well. Depending on their proximity, you may have different obstacles to deal with in this area.

If your grandchildren are far away, or at least more than a few hours' drive, you'll have to plan your vacation time to maximize the time you can spend with them. This will take a bit of balancing, because you have to respect the parents' (your child and their spouse's) expectations and needs for this new little one. Remember that they will hold their own ideas about how they want their schedule to go. It is your job to fit into this, not disrupt it. Be a willing listener, compromise, and try to respect their desires.

If your grandchildren are in close proximity, separate challenges may arise. You'll want to give your children the space and time to get their routines figured out, but also be there to help when necessary. Everyone loves to spoil their grandchildren, and you can; just be mindful of the parents. You still need to instill and reinforce manners and morals, just as you did with your child as they grew up.

This is the time to ensure that your grandchild is off to a good start in life as far as health goes. The most important thing you can do is show them love, and when it comes to eating, set a good example. Have healthful foods around for them to eat when they visit. Plan fun activities that keep your grandchildren active and make them think.

15
LAST DAYS

Only one thing in life is for certain: we are all going to die someday. This is not something to fear, but instead something to respect. I hope that by the time you arrive at the later stages of life, you are satisfied with your journey. If you have been taking care of yourself by balancing your inner and outer circles, you should be entering this part of your life peacefully, not painfully.

If all goes well, you should be able to plan this stage of your life. Even people who get sick due to unhealthy habits throughout their lives usually have the opportunity to plan. I think it is much better to be able to make your plan and ensure that your family knows your desires before you are on your deathbed.

I learned this idea of planning when my father was dying. Although I was only eleven years old, I could see that he was planning. From the time he was diagnosed with cancer, both of my parents were clear about how he wanted things to go. At first, these plans involved treatments, and attempts to make our lives as normal as possible. Later, they transitioned to ensuring that our future would be as good as it could possibly be. Finally, things ended with requests that people come to visit him in hospice. My father asked my mother to contact people and tell them to be there within a certain amount of time; and when that time was up, he passed away.

Everyone's plan is different, but don't be afraid to think and talk about these things. Make your desires known. Some discussions might center around what to do if you are hospitalized or in a vegetative state. You may also want to express your desires, hopes, and dreams for your loved ones. Whatever is important to you, express it, and have the conversation; then you can be at peace during the last days of your life rather than stressed or panicked. This will also allow others to accept your death more easily and naturally.

16
CONCLUSIONS

Your life can be viewed as a history of the choices you made, and the repercussions of those choices. Balancing your inner and outer circles influences your choices, and can impart a positive effect upon your life as a whole.

First, you must understand what makes up your inner and outer circles; then you have to balance these two areas in order to maximize health. Remember that everyone is different, and they will deal with their inner and outer circles differently, as well. Your circles, however, will inevitably overlap with those of others, leaving an imprint and influence each time.

Staying healthy is not so difficult if you honestly consider and address the things affecting your outer and inner circles. This book goes through the different phases of life, making suggestions for each one. As far as eating goes, it is actually pretty simple: try to eat well about 90% of the time. When you are eating well, have as many vegetables and fruits as you want. Eat lean meats, nuts, beans, and legumes. Choose whole grains, and eat organic whenever possible. Eat very few processed foods. Try to cook at home.

Start your family out early eating the foods listed above, teach your children about being healthy, and continue to learn and research on your own. Don't forget to exercise at least five days a week.

17
QUICK TIPS

Inner Circle

- Environment

    - Always conscious of what you are put-ting on your body (creams, deodorant, make-up) and choose things with the least amounts of harmful chemicals

    - Put yourself in the most positive envi-ronment possible

- Eating Out

    - Ascertain the healthiest choices and combinations from what is available on the menu

- Don't be afraid to ask that items to be prepared in a healthier way
- Shopping
- Buy organic whenever possible
- Shop around the perimeter of the grocery store
- Read labels
  - Avoid artificial sweeteners (aspartame, sucralose, asulfame K, and saccharin, to name a few)
  - Avoid bad fats (trans fats, partially hydrogenated oils, and saturated fats) and increase good fats
  - Avoid GMOs
  - Avoid artificial colors (any color with a number after it, such as Red 40)
  - Avoid added sugar (by any name)
- Cook Once, Eat Twice
- Remember Michael Pollan's advice: "Eat (good) food. Not too much. Mostly plants.
  - Everyone is busy; make a little more of some meals, and save the leftovers for the next day

Outer Circle

- Personal Outlook

    - Remain positive

    - Don't succumb to jealousy

    - Remember that things can always be worse, and that we never know the full extent of what another may be going through

    - Anger only leads to poor health—not resolution

    - Cultivate confidence

    - Practice gratitude

    - Put love first

- You Can Do It!

    - Don't doubt yourself

    - Don't let others bring you down

    - Remember Abraham Lincoln: never fear failure

- Stress

  - Balance your outer circle

  - Find ways to cope with stress (exercise, talking, hobbies, etc.)

- Entertainment

  - Find healthy ways to have fun

  - Engage your mind and body

- Relationships

  - Resolve relationships that act as poor contributors to your health in a manageable, healthy way

  - Surround yourself with supportive relationships

  - Pets are therapeutic

  - Communicate, communicate, communicate!

- Career

  - Try to do what you like for a living; or take action to get there

- Seek out, and contribute to, positive work environments

- Finances

    - Save

    - Budget

    - Don't worry about what others have

- Spirituality

    - Religious activities

    - Non-religious activities

    - Cultivate a sense of deeper meaning

- Physical Environment

    - Mitigate allergens

    - Avoid pollution

    - Avoid insecticides and pesticides

    - Use environmentally responsible cleaning and skin care products

- Exercise

    - Contributes to a healthy weight

- Allows body systems to work more efficiently

- Improves mood

- Reduces stress

- Contributes to better health in the latter part of life

- Linkages

  - Knowledge-get it!

  - Awareness-have it!

  - Motivation-use it!

  - Make the changes to your inner and outer circle that lead to a healthier life

  - Make your healthy lifestyle contagious and be an example to others